How to Find Happiness

by Sri Swami Satchidananda

Library of Congress Cataloging in
Publication Data
Satchidananda, Swami.
How to Find Happiness

I. Title.
2011
ISBN 978-0-932040-46-6

Printed in the United States of America.

Integral Yoga® Publications
Satchidananda Ashram–Yogaville, Inc.
108 Yogaville Way, Buckingham, VA, USA 23921
www.YogaAndPeace.org

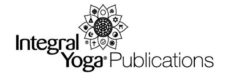

Yogaville, Virginia, USA

Books & Booklets by
Sri Swami Satchidananda

Beyond Words

Enlightening Tales

The Golden Present

Bound To Be Free:
The Liberating Power
of Prison Yoga

The Healthy Vegetarian

Heaven on Earth

Integral Yoga Hatha

Kailash Journal

The Living Gita

To Know Your Self

Yoga Sutras of Patanjali

Titles in this special
Peter Max cover art series:

Meditation

The Key to Peace

Overcoming Obstacles

Adversity and Awakening

Satchidananda Sutras

Gems of Wisdom

Pathways to Peace

How to Find Happiness

The Be-Attitudes

Everything Will Come to You

Thou Art That:
How to Know Yourself

Free Yourself

The Guru Within

Books/Films about
Sri Swami Satchidananda

The Master's Touch

Sri Swami Satchidananda:
   Apostle of Peace

Sri Swami Satchidananda:
   Portrait of a Modern Sage

Boundless Giving: The Life and Service of
Sri Swami Satchidananda

Living Yoga: The life and teachings of
   Swami Satchidananda

Many Paths, One Truth: The Interfaith
   Message of Swami Satchidananda

The Essence of Yoga:
   The Path of Integral Yoga with
   Swami Satchidananda

For complete listing of books, CDs and DVDs:
www.iydbooks.com

Dedication

The teachings of Sri Gurudev Swami Satchidananda are universal. Not limited to any one organization, religion or country, Sri Gurudev received invitations from around the world to speak about the way to peace–individual and global.

At every moment, we have the opportunity to be a part of a positive evolution in the world. Though we always have challenges to face in life, we should never lose our hope for individual happiness and for world peace. The vision and the teachings of Sri Gurudev focus on the inherent unity in our apparent diversity. As a global family, the common bond that we share is our spiritual nature.

This small book was originally presented as a humble offering to our beloved Gurudev on the joyous occasion of his 76th *Jayanthi* (birth anniversary) in 1990. It is now re-designed and re-dedicated to Sri Gurudev, to his vision of peace and unity and to the seekers of all faiths in their search for true and lasting happiness.

May peace and happiness, love and light pervade the entire universe. *OM Shanti*.

Acknowledgments

How To Find Happiness was compiled from articles by Sri Gurudev that have appeared over the years in *Integral Yoga Magazine*, a vehicle for spreading the love, light and wisdom of Sri Gurudev to Yoga students worldwide for over forty years. Integral Yoga Magazine is a highly valued link for those who do not have the opportunity to visit Satchidananda Ashram as often as they would like.

This booklet was originally published in French, having been compiled by Mitra Schmidt of Integral Yoga France. We would like to offer our thanks to Mitra for the original text, which was entitled, *A La Recherche Du Bonheur*.

Our love and gratitude to pop artist icon Peter Max. His art, which defined a generation, is instantly recognizable and continues to inspire. Peter Max is the person who first hosted Sri Swami Satchidananda in America, and it's a privilege to have his artwork gracing the cover of this special series of small gift books. Also, we're so thankful to Victor Arjuna Zurbel for all his graphic design talents and for his work with

Peter Atman Max in bringing this series to fruition. Special thanks as well to Reverend Kumari de Sachy for her editing skills and for all her dedicated Karma Yoga. Our thanks to Reverend Prem Anjali for overseeing the production of this book series.

We also wish to thank the Harry Wadhwani family, the Prakash and Mahesh Daswani families, and Reverend Sivani Alderman, whose generous donations made this and other publications possible.

Contents

A Pure Heart

Yoga means tranquility of mind and flexibility of body. The *Bible* presents this as purity of heart. Talking about the only needed quality to see God, the *Bible* says, "Blessed are the pure in heart, for they shall see God." Whoever is pure in heart shall see God. It doesn't say whoever built temples or churches, whoever printed thousands of scriptures or burned any amount of candles every Sunday.

It's immaterial whether you do those things or not. If you do them, it's all right. But what is the ultimate requirement to see God? Purity of heart. And that's Yoga. That's religion. And that should be our life. Our faith and Yoga need not be different from our day-to-day lives.

Just by going to church every Sunday, you cannot become a Christian; it's not the going alone that does it. What should happen? What is the reason to attend religious services? You attend religious services to clean your heart. Why do we light candles in a service or meditation? To bring forth the Light within, or, at least to remember that we should realize that Light. All rituals, practices, services or various types of worship are aimed toward keeping the heart clean.

The *Bible* uses a beautiful term, "the heart," which stands for the physical as well as the mental heart. If you say somebody is a kind-hearted person, or a soft-hearted person, you don't just put your finger there to see how soft the heart is. If you call somebody your "sweetheart," do you actually taste the heart? No. The word "heart" stands for both the physical and the subtle-body as well as for the mind. It's a pretty word. In one word, they are trying to tell us two things: let your physical heart be clean and, also, let your mental heart be clean. Blessed are the pure in heart, physically and mentally.

The physical heart represents the entire body. In a way, the entire body gets its nourishment from the heart. The heart supplies everything; it's the heart of the person, so keep it clean. Stay away from anything that would adversely affect your physical heart. That's why we recommend certain restrictions in what we eat and drink. We also recommend clean air and proper exercise. At the same time, we recommend not to over-exercise. The heart

needs exercise, but it should no‿
capacity.

Unfortunately, in the n‿
of the important ideas that on‿
various religions have been someho‿
or comfortably forgotten. If you read the‿
sages and saints of all religions, almost every ‿
talked about the importance of eating clean food.
To be more precise, most recommended clean,
vegetarian food. They never recommended meat,
liquor or alcohol. And we, in the name of Yoga,
are trying to bring back those teachings again.

Unfortunately, we do many things in our
lives that are bad for us. In fact, even when they
know that it's bad, people still do it; and then,
they find it hard to get out of that bad habit, to
stay away from it. To prove this point, take a
census and let the whole world answer your
question: "Is smoking good for you?" Let the
answer come from their hearts.

Without a doubt, they will all say, "No, it's
not necessary. It's not good for my health. It's not
good for my lungs or for my heart." They all
know that, including the person who paid a huge

of money for a big poster that declares, rally Refreshes You." Let that person touch r her heart and tell you whether a cigarette going to refresh you naturally. It's not true. And we all know that.

Furthermore, that's an important point to be noted. For we all know what is right and what is wrong, but many don't seem to have the strength to stay away from those things. In order for us to follow the right and stay away from the wrong, we have to build up our strength. Our minds must be really strong. When you say, "I don't want to touch this anymore," you should be able to stay away from that. You should be able to forget it. If somebody brings it to you tomorrow, you may not even recognize what it is. For instance, suppose you say, "I'm not going to smoke. I don't want cigarettes anymore. I'm forgetting cigarettes." And then, if the next day, somebody offers a cigarette, you'll say, "What is this stick?" It's as though you completely erased that form and name from your brain.

And this applies to any harmful habit. You could do it if you develop your will. Developing the will is very important. That is where concentration and meditation come in; they enable you to strengthen the mind. We all know the proverb, "As you think, so you become." If you keep on thinking of something, you are going to realize that, because–through the thinking of it–the mind gets so strong that it's able to accomplish what it wants. Then again, in order to strengthen the mind, we should understand why it is weak. How does that weakness happen?

To understand this process, let's take an imaginary trip to a physics lab or try some mechanical engineering. Take a large tank and fill it up with water. The tank has nine or ten big taps all around, but when you fill the tank with water, you fail to close all the taps. So you keep on filling. You wanted to build up some pressure in one tap, but all the water keeps flowing out. How could you build up the pressure in that one tap? It's simple. Just close off the rest of the taps. Call it physics or mechanical engineering or anything.

In any case, when you close all the other taps, you get the maximum pressure from the remaining tap. The water tank can be several stories high, but the minute you open a couple of taps the pressure comes down, and the level of the water won't reach that high. In the same way, this is how the mind functions. You simultaneously open the tap of the mind in a hundred areas, and in each area, you see the mind going, but without force. The level has just simply dropped.

Certainly, you want to achieve everything, but not at the same time. So, close all the channels. Open the one channel that you want to be predominant—that is concentration. It's simple. You are blocking your mind from going into all channels and directing it to one channel, to one thing. Your concentration can be on an object, an idea, a prayer or a mantra. And, of course, the mind has a tendency to run toward all the other channels. Therefore, every time you see it running to another channel, turn the tap tight. Train the mind to run through only one tap.

You can achieve that level of concentration if you train the mind. But don't think that the minute you sit for concentration you'll be able to do it overnight. It takes a while, because the mind got used to running here and there in hundreds of directions. So, gently block the way; you don't need to be rough and rude with the mind. Be nice, as a mother would train a baby: "Oh, my sweet, that's not the way. Just do it this way, then I'll give you a treat."

Our motive is not to break the mind, but to train it. The mind is like a wild horse. It's like a restless monkey. You can train it, but be patient. Yes, it might be difficult to achieve, but it's worth it. You, yourself, can do it. The spiritual teacher can only guide you, give you all the methods to try. Your success depends upon how sincere you are, how serious you are.

According to Bhagavan Patanjali, to get the benefit of Yoga you have to practice for a long time, without break and with total interest. And when will the Yoga practices help you? When you are tired of everything else. When you have tried all those things and know that they're not going to help you anymore, you can renounce them. A person who has come to that realization is called a spiritual seeker.

In the yogic life, if you know why you are doing it, you will enjoy everything–however difficult it may be. That's very important. In fact, that is yogic action. A yogi will perform everything to enjoy. The whole life is a joy for the yogi. If it's going to be a life of suffering, why would you even want to be a yogi? In fact, it's a yogi who really enjoys life, because he or she knows how to live it, how to enjoy it without getting caught in it.

Of course, that way of thinking doesn't happen overnight. In the beginning you might get a little tense, thinking, "I must do this. I must do that. Otherwise, I won't attain my goal." When you think that way, even in the name of Yoga practices, you lose the little peace that you do have.

So, keep reminding yourself: "It's for the peace that I'm doing everything. If the very doing itself is going to disturb my peace, either the doing is wrong or my approach is wrong." Yoga means peace and serenity of mind. The mind should always be peaceful, serene, calm and clean. When that happens, you'll know the ultimate benefit. So just remember: It's worth it.

How to Succeed in Yoga

Yoga means to control the mind, to master the mind. Patanjali's *Yoga Sutras* begins by saying: "Control of thoughts is Yoga–*Yoga chitta vritti nirodhah*." (*Sutra* 1.2) But how is it to be done? Even the ideal disciple, Arjuna, says to Sri Krishna in the *Bhagavad Gita*, "My mind is verily restless, turbulent and obstinate. I deem it as hard to control as the wind." (*Gita*, 6.34)

Here, Krishna makes a very helpful point: "By practice and non-attachment, the mind can be controlled." (*Gita*, 6.35) This very same clue is also given by Sri Patanjali in his *Yoga Sutras*: "*Abhyasa vairagyaabhyaam nirodhah*." (*Sutra* 1.12) *Abhyasa* and *vairagya* mean practice and non-attachment, respectively.

Krishna and Patanjali are referring to continuous practice, not just one day a week or five minutes in the morning or evening and the rest of the time you just do anything you want. No; the aim must be kept always. It's something like meditating for five or ten minutes in the morning, five minutes in the evening and then just leaving the mind uncontrolled and allowing it to go where it wants during the rest of the day. Or, like holding the rudder for only ten minutes and then just leaving it uncontrolled, letting the wind toss the boat any way it wants. By doing that you won't reach the shore.

When you see a boat or a big ship, what is the most important thing there? It's the captain standing in front of the compass in order to navigate the vessel. You set your boat to a particular degree, a particular direction. If it's 180 degrees, then you go completely straight, always 180 degrees. You may say, "Oh, I'm just a couple of degrees off; it doesn't matter." But where will you end up? You may say, "I missed by only one or two degrees," but, at the end, the distance is really great.

That is why constant attention, awareness and vigilance are necessary. Somebody has to be holding the wheel, watching the compass. Is it going in the right direction or not? If by any chance you make a mistake, if you get caught by the wind, then you correct your course. The navigator must immediately work out the course correction. Either in a ship or a plane, without that course correction, you can never reach the destination. If you start in New York and want to end up in Los Angeles, probably you'll end up in Miami!

Particularly if you read a little bit about flying, you see that there are so many things involved in it: tailwind, headwind, crosswind, temperature changes. You have to calculate all these elements in order to see that your plane flies in the right direction. It's a beautiful lesson. Just to fly a plane, we need all these things. What about this plane, the body? Here also, we have headwind, tailwind, crosswind, turbulence, how many things! And, if a big plane flies close by, you get great disturbance, you get pulled. So, you have to be constantly at it.

I'm going to tell you a story to illustrate this point. Once upon a time, there were two boatmen. They knew how to row, but they didn't own a boat. One day, they wanted to steal a boat in order to go to a neighboring town on the river Ganges. So, around midnight, they went to the shore and found a rowboat.

They were really well prepared. What kind of preparation did they have? They had plenty of gasoline–for themselves! Of course, rowboats don't need gasoline, but the rowers may need it.

What I mean is, the boatmen were drunk! They had plenty of high octane gasoline. They had really filled up the tank, so they were walking slowly. You can imagine how they were walking. They got down to the river, and the minute they saw the boat, they were so happy: "Ah, we got a boat–come on, get in." Then, they found the oars and started rowing. They were just singing a song and rowing the boat.

All night, they were rowing; and, slowly the dawn finally came. As you may know, people normally come to the Ganges in the early morning to take a bath. The two boatmen saw a couple of people coming, but, surprisingly, the faces were familiar. "That's strange," they thought. "How did they get here so easily? We have been rowing half the night." Then, by the time it was a little more clear, they began seeing familiar buildings.

"Hey," they said to the bathers. "We're still in the same place. What happened?"

Then the bathers asked, "Why? Why are you wondering what happened? What did you want to do? Whose boat is this?"

"Oh, no, no. We just wanted to go to the neighboring town and come back soon. We've been rowing the whole night. I don't know why we're still here."

"Why you're still here? You fools! You forgot to undo the knot. All the while, you were tied to the shore." No doubt, they had been practicing, months and months and months of practice. "Oh, I did all the *japa*. I did all the *pranayama*. I went to all the Gurus. I practiced every technique." Unfortunately they were still tied down. They didn't detach from the anchor.

See? Mere practice alone is not enough. Let us know that positively. You must have that dispassion, which is called *vairagya* or non-attachment. I don't say that those practices are no good. In a way, it's better than doing nothing. At least, instead of going to a bar, you're hearing about Yoga. Likewise, if the boatment hadn't been rowing all night in the boat, they would have been in the gambling den. So, practice is an advantage, no doubt.

But you can't reach the shore, that is, you can't attain the goal, unless the bondages are removed.

Unfortunately, in our boats, we don't have only one anchor–there are thousands of anchors everywhere. Everything that you call "mine, mine, mine" is holding you. That's why I say that if you want to know how far away you are from your goal–call it God or peace–I can give you an easy method with which you can check the distance. The easiest way is to gather some paper and start writing down everything that you call "mine:" *my* house, *my* body, *my* brain, *my* intelligence, *my* child, *my* wife, *my* money, *my* race, *my* country, *my* this, *my* that.

List everything that you can call "mine;" don't omit even one thing. If the list is really long, it means that you're that far away from your goal. If you can reduce the list, then you're coming closer. If there's nothing for you to write as "mine," then you're there already. That's all. It's very simple. You don't need to practice anything. You don't even need to practice any other Yoga.

This is the essence. If you really want to get peace, the simplest way is to make a check: "How many mines have I put around me?" The more mines around you, the more you are in trouble. Every "mine" is ready to explode! You're making your whole life a war field, throwing "mines" everywhere. So, if you've already thrown them, call a good minesweeper–the Guru. Mine-sweeper (or mind-sweeper), he or she will know how to take away the fuse. And, once the fuse is taken away, there won't be confusion. And how will the Guru take the fuse out? Just by just changing the label, by taking the label away from all that you call "mine, mine, mine," replacing it with "Thine, Thine, Thine."

What I mean by that is that then you are developing dispassion. You are not attached to things. You can keep them around, but don't call them "mine." Imagine that they have given me a chair to sit in and give a talk. Imagine that it's a very comfortable chair, like a throne. I could even say it is my seat, as long as I'm sitting in it. But when the lecture is over, I can't take it with me and leave. It's only been given to me to use during my talk. Likewise, everything, even your body, is given to you for your use, not just to pamper it, constantly standing in front of the mirror for one and a half hours and patching everything up. No. Use it; don't misuse it.

To make another analogy, suppose a vehicle is given to you. You have to take good care of it.

You need to put the proper fuel in it. If the vehicle is made to use high octane, don't put crude oil into it. See that every nut and bolt is properly tightened—neither too tight nor too loose. Sometimes, people themselves get too tight or too loose. Either way, too tight or too loose, there will be trouble.

Again, everything in life is given to you for your use, not to own, not to possess. And that is what you call dispassion or detachment. Moreover, when you use anything, you have a responsibility to keep it clean, to use it properly. The responsibility is there. Don't think that because it's not yours, you can just do anything to it or leave it. You're still responsible.

This kind of detachment should be understood properly. You can't become irresponsible, just leaving everything and running away. If you do, wherever you go, you'll still be attached to something. If you're not attached to your mansion, within a few weeks you'll be attached to your teepee.

What does it matter? It makes no difference if it's a mansion or a teepee. It doesn't matter whether it's your nice suit, hat, tie and coat, or all the bleached-out or worn-out jeans. How many people are attached even to those worn-out jeans? What's the idea behind all the bleached-out jeans? Clothing is something to cover the body with, that's all. It should be neat and clean. That attitude toward clothing is not going to bind you, as long as you're not attached to it and don't go to the other extreme.

Finally, unless there's non-attachment, practices will not bring much result. Side by side, there should be *abhyasa* and *vairagya*–practice and non-attachment. They are the two wings of the bird, and both are necessary. With the help of these two wings, let your soul soar high to bring you perfect mastery over your own mind, to enjoy perfect peace and joy always.

Selflessness and Karma Yoga

Perfection in action is Yoga. A yogi can sit well, talk well, eat well, sleep well and enjoy things without getting caught up in them. A yogi can enjoy the world, because he or she knows the limitations, knows how far to go. Who are the good surfers? Those who can ride the big waves. Because they know that they're not going to get caught, yogis will even watch for big waves. They have surfboards and know how to balance themselves on them. Balance means tranquil.

If you have a balanced mind, that's your surfboard. You're steady on it. Whatever wave comes, you just go out and enjoy it without getting caught. You're in the world, but never of the world. This means that Integral Yoga embraces the entire life from morning until evening. Everything should be yogic, from the minute you start brushing your teeth to the minute you go to bed. Do it well, and do it now.

Karma Yoga, the path of selfless service, is the best form of Yoga. Even if you don't have time to meditate, to do asanas, to eat or to sleep, it doesn't matter. If you have an opportunity to do Karma Yoga, do that first. Through Karma Yoga your heart, mind and body will be soon cleaned. Here you'll see your limitations and drawbacks, not in your meditation. During Karma Yoga, you'll come to understand your attitudes and moods, not when you are all alone. So, test yourself in the field.

Karma Yoga means a selfless act. If you're motivated to do something for others and don't expect any personal results or reward, such an action is called Karma Yoga. But if you expect any result for your benefit, then it is merely karma. It's just a labor: "I do this so that I can get that." But true Karma Yoga is service performed for the joy of serving. You don't even wait for a thanks. That way, you can keep your mind calm, without any disturbance.

Whether people appreciate your action or not, even if they criticize you, that's their business. You've done your job to your capacity. You're satisfied with what you've done and don't expect anything in return, so your mind is always calm. That is Yoga—calmness of mind. If you keep calm during the karma, it's Karma Yoga. If you get disturbed during your action, it's karma.

The *Bhagavad Gita* says, "All that you are entitled to is to act. Just do, but don't wait for the result." Because when you wait for the result, you build tension and become upset. If you don't get the result, you're frustrated and angry; if you do get the result, you become greedy. Even if you don't want more, you still want to protect what you have, because you feel that having will make you happy. You're afraid of losing the possession, because your happiness seems to depend on that possession.

The fear of losing is always waiting, and in order to be more happy you want more things. Then, if anybody puts up a barrier to prevent you from accumulating, you'll hate that person. Your own selfishness causes hatred, fear, jealousy and anger.

On the other hand, if you don't want anything from anybody, then you're freed from these tendencies. That's why Karma Yoga will relieve you from all this strain. You are always happy, always peaceful. But *karmi*s are those who are interested only in the outcome. Even the mere thought of the outcome makes them so excited that they lose everything.

If we only knew how to act—not waiting for the result, without any selfishness—we wouldn't lose our happiness or our peace. Do anything you want. Even your personal eating may seem that you're doing it for your own sake: you're tasting it; you're filling the stomach. Is it not karma, then? No, it isn't. When you want to take the car on the road, you have to fill up the tank. Your body is the same. Even when you eat and drink, it's not for your sake; it's so that you can serve others.

Karma Yogis work with more zeal than ordinary people because they're doing it as a service to God, they have more interest than people who work just for their own benefit. If you're cooking your dinner, it can be anything. But if you cook for some honored guest, then you want to offer nicer items. The plates will be well polished. You'll take out all your special dishes and silverware. Why? Because there's a joy in doing something as an offering, and you'll never get that joy when you do it just for yourself.

Many, unfortunately, have never tasted that joy. It's unforgettable. If you really do something for somebody else and experience that joy, you will never want to do something for yourself.

You'll always look for opportunities to serve. It's even sort of selfish—because you miss that joy, whether it is day or night. It's something sweet and delicious. And that's what's called a dedicated life. There's supreme joy in it.

Once a month or once in two months, try to set aside some time and say, "This is my Karma Yoga week. The whole week, I should be totally selfless. I won't be doing anything for my sake." Or, choose just one day, like when you choose a fasting day, and say to yourself, "This is a selfless day." Karma Yoga is give, give, give. Don't worry about how you'll manage to survive.

If people know that you're here to give, and if you're really giving, it's their business, and in their best interest, to keep you well. If a tree is always giving a lot of fruit, won't the gardener take special care of the tree? He or she won't forget to water it daily and may even put a fence around it. Not that the tree demanded anything; it just did its duty.

In the same way, if your life is useful to people, they'll take care of you. On the other hand, if you're not useful, why should you even live? There's no need. So, wherever you are, just give joyfully. It's true that you may not get proper care immediately. But forget it, and it will come.

When nature, the Cosmic Consciousness, knows fully well that you're really offering your service and not expecting anything in return, once that is proved, then abundance will be with you. That selfless life is what you call God. God was never selfish. And God's Nature was never selfish. So, if you lead a selfless life, you are in God. And when you have God, certainly everything else will be added unto you.

Ishvara Pranidhana: Self-Surrender

The practice of *Ishvara pranidhana* is simple but great. It's surrendering to the Supreme Being. I understand this to mean dedicating the fruits of your actions to God or to humanity–God in manifestation. Dedicate everything, your study, your *japa* (mantra repetition) and your practices, to God. When you give such things, God accepts them but then gives them back many times magnified. You never lose what you've given. Even virtuous, meritorious deeds will bind you in some form or other if you do them with an egoistic feeling. Therefore, every time you do something feel, "May this be dedicated to God." If you constantly remember to do this, the mind will be free and tranquil. Try not to possess anything for yourself. Temporarily keep things but feel that you are just a trustee, not an owner.

Be like the mother who receives a soul, nourishes it for nine months and then lets it come out into the world. If the mother were always to keep the baby in her womb, what would happen? There would be great pain. Once something has ripened, it should be passed on. So dedication is true Yoga. Say, "I am Thine.

All is Thine. Thy will be done." "Mine" binds; "Thine" liberates. If you drop "mines" all over, they will undermine your life or blow up in your face. But if you change all the "mines" to "Thine," you'll always be safe. So let us dedicate our lives for the sake of the entire humanity. Every minute, every breath, every atom of our bodies should repeat this mantra: "dedication, dedication, giving, giving, loving, loving." That is the best *japa*, the best Yoga that will bring us all permanent peace and joy and keep the mind free from the disturbances of the thought waves.

Ishvara pranidhana is a life of dedication, of offering everything to God or to humanity. Why do I add humanity? When we want to offer something to God, where and who is God? Is God sitting somewhere waiting for us to give something? God made the world out of God. The world itself is God. All that's outside of us is God. When we dedicate our lives to the benefit of humanity, we've dedicated ourselves to God. Whatever we do can easily be transformed into worship by our attitude. We can do anything and everything as long as we do it with the idea of serving the world at large. We can serve our tables, our chairs, and everything around us. If we don't pull chairs mercilessly from one corner to another, we're serving them. If we drag them, they cry. Anything handled roughly will feel pain. There should be a gentle, yogic touch with everything—even our spoons, forks and plates.

When you pray, it shouldn't be to ask for this and for that. Your prayer is to be used by the Cosmic Plan. That's why in prayer we say, "I am Thine. All is Thine. Thy will be done." You shouldn't demand, "Give me a little of this, a little of that." Some people do pray that way, but how do they know if it's going to help them? Sometimes, you may ask for something that will not help you; it may even hurt you. The sincere prayer is one in which you don't demand anything from God. You just say, "God, you know what is good for me. I'm your child. Guide me. Direct me." On the other hand, even without your asking, God is going to take care of you, no doubt. But if you feel like asking, say, "Mother, I'm yours. You do anything you want." If you still want to add something, say, "Let me have this kind of understanding always: that I am Your child, that You are taking care of me every minute. Let me not forget this. Give me the boon of constantly remembering this truth."

I can't tell you how to surrender. You'll know when to surrender. When everything else fails and when there is no other way then you give up. Surrendering means to give up, isn't that so? And when will you give up? When you are positive that nothing is going to save you. When you realize that, surrender comes. However, if you have even a little faith in your own capacity, it's not complete surrender.

This point is beautifully presented in a story from the great epic the *Mahabharata*. Through gambling, the husband of the princess Draupadi lost her to another man. The winner, the other man, wanted to shame Draupadi's husband and family. In those days, when you wanted to show that you had victory over someone, you did something damaging to that person's reputation. So, he had Draupadi brought to the center of the room, and he tried to pull off Draupadi's *sari*. According to the conditions of the game, her husband couldn't do anything about it, so she couldn't expect help from her husband or from anyone else. She realized that the only way was to pray to Lord Krishna: "Krishna, Krishna, Krishna, please come help me. I am in a difficult situation," she called. All the while, she held tight to her *sari*.

By the way, do you know how a *sari* is worn? Out of one long piece of cloth, there is an upper cloth and three or four rounds tied around the waist and wrapped over a slip. Anyway, the fellow had the upper cloth in his hand, and he was pulling the *sari*. One round came off. The second round came off. Still, Draupadi held tight and called "Krishna! Krishna!" But no help came. So she held up one hand to Krishna, but kept the other hand holding the *sari*. Still, no help came and, still, he pulled. Finally, there was only one more round of cloth left. That's all. (Of course, if that round comes off, it would be the end of the story!)

So, Draupadi realizing her predicament, cried: "My God, I couldn't help myself. I've already lost two rounds of the *sari* by trying to do it myself. If I lose this final round, I'll be doomed." It was at that moment that it dawned on her: "What am I doing? I can't take care of myself anymore."

With that realization, she simply let go of the *sari* and lifted both hands up to call: "Krishna! You are the only refuge for me. If you want me to face this, okay. I totally trust you. You are my sole refuge. Krishna!" She had both hands raised, and that fellow was pulling and pulling on the *sari*. He had thought that he had the last round of cloth, but the cloth kept coming. And he kept pulling, and yards and yards and yards of the *sari* came. Finally, he got tired. He couldn't pull anymore. He gave up, and Draupadi was saved.

This story illustrates that even God can't come and help you as long as you have faith in your own strength. In that case, you're not totally surrendered, and God says, "Okay, just take care of yourself." There are hundreds and hundreds of stories to illustrate this point. In the *Bible*, didn't a woman simply touch the garment of Lord Jesus and get cured? What cured her? Jesus said, "You had faith. It's not my garment; your faith cured you." All the scriptures say the same thing. That's what you call surrender. If you have implicit faith and trust in God, you'll feel, "I have surrendered myself to God. No harm will come to me. God will take care of me every minute, in every way." And you will be taken care of.

Unfortunately, an unclean mind can never harbor such faith. It will come and go, come and go. So, we have to clean our minds in our daily life so that the faith can grow, can get well rooted. Fortunate are the people who have that kind of faith.

The Safest, Simplest and Happiest Life

If you put yourself totally in God's hands,
every one of you can do much more in your life.
Give up your ego. Give up the feeling that, "I can
do this." That feeling really comes and interferes
with everything. Instead, think, "Let God function
through me."

Of all the *slokas* in the *Bhagavad Gita,* one
sloka is called the supreme, the gem, the essence.
It comes almost toward the end of the *Bhagavad
Gita.* And it simply says: "Just give up everything.
Renounce everything. Even your will, your
ego, your intelligence, your foolishness, your
everything." Yes, everything should be given
up. Not just simple renunciation. It should be
complete renunciation of everything.

In *The Living Gita,* we translate this as:
"Renounce all duties (*dharma*), and just come
to Me for refuge. I will take you beyond sin and
guilt, where there is neither grief nor sorrow."
What a wonderful saying. Renounce all actions,
all duties; completely give up. Lord Krishna says,
"Surrender yourself to Me. Know that I am the
only one who does everything, who takes care of

everything. I am the only refuge, the sole refuge." If you do that, "I'll free you from all troubles, all problems, all your sins, virtues, whatever it is." He also says, "Don't doubt," because He knows the human mind. Having heard all this, still, you might say, "Ahh, maybe it's all just philosophy." God knows how the human mind works, so, lastly, He says, "Don't doubt please. I assure you." Literally, He says, "I promise you this because you are my beloved."

In the beginning of the *Bhagavad Gita*, Arjuna exhausts all his arguments and intellectual gymnastics. He asks, "Why should I do all this? Why can't I keep quiet? Should I fight when it's for a just cause?" He lists all the reasons not to do anything. "I just want to cop out, give up, and run away to a cave. What good are all these things? What good is it to save all these people or to kill all those so-called evil people? I didn't bring them; I'm not going to take them. It's not my duty."

That beautiful, mischievous God, in the form of Lord Krishna, just watched him and smiled, "Okay, come on, come on; empty it all out. Anything more?" He simply nodded and smiled as Arjuna talked. At last, Arjuna realized that he was simply talking, that's all. He was creating sounds for argument. The argument was not sound. He felt ashamed. Finally, Arjuna said, "What a fool I am. I'm blabbering, exhausting my intelligence. Why can't I do the simplest thing? Okay, Lord, that's it. I'm falling at Your feet; I surrender at Your feet. That's it. You do whatever you want; it's none of my business. I didn't create the world, and I'm not going to save it or destroy it. It's Your job. You did it. You created everything; You created me too. You know what You are doing; please do it. I'm Your disciple."

Then, the whole *Bhagavad Gita* starts. Toward the end, Lord Krishna says this: "Give up everything. Become my instrument. Let me do whatever I really feel is right. Let me work through you. Then, you don't become responsible for anything, and I can make the best use of you." That is the beauty of giving up into the hands of God. Very simply, the saint Avvaiyar said, "Renounce all wants, and you are Home." If you give up all your "I," "me," "mine," you're already liberated.

You have freedom. You don't even have to write a constitution. The best constitution is to surrender everything to God. It's really very simple to do. Remember, it's easy to give up things; it's hard to hold onto them. With that holding on, comes a lot of anxiety, worry, fear, jealousy and on and on.

Another great saint said, "Lord, I don't mind what you do with me. People may give their opinions. Some may say "right;" some may say "wrong." Should I worry? You are the one who is handling it all. You drive anywhere you want. Go to the movie, fine; go to the nightclub, fine; go to the church, fine. You're the one behind the wheel; You're the driver. And if You get into trouble, they don't punish me, the car; You're the culprit." You can't say, "The car took me to the nightclub. The car took me to rob the bank. Charge the car." No. The driver is responsible, not the driven. That's the driving force behind everything.

I'm just telling you what I know, what I followed in my own life. If you like it, take it, try it. It's very simple. With this attitude of surrender, everything falls into place. Why should you hate anybody? Why should you dislike anybody? Everybody is good; everybody is wonderful; everybody is the instrument of God. God is working through everybody, not only through you. When you give up, you know that. You see God's hand in everything, every face. If somebody comes and blames you, it's God. If somebody comes and praises you, it's God. The moment you know that God is working through you, you see the same hand working through everything. You see everyone with equal vision. Automatically, you begin to love everybody as you would love yourself. The entire nature is That. "Without God's force, not even an atom moves." Everything moves like that. We are all being moved.

Let God do whatever is necessary. Who are you even to let God do something? God does it anyway and doesn't wait for your permission. We say, "God, do whatever You want." God doesn't say, "Oh, okay. Only now that I got your permission will I do what I want." See how the ego sneaks into everything? As if to say, "I am permitting You; You can do whatever You want now," and until then, God was waiting. No; God was already doing it.

You'll have the safest and the simplest and the happiest life if you surrender in this way. Otherwise, your ego is in everything: "Oh, I should have taken care of that. I should have done this. I'm responsible for that. I have to get something for those people." I, I, I. Aye, aye, aye!

Then again, surrender doesn't simply mean that you don't do anything, that you go to your room and lie down. When God prompts you to do something, do it. And remember, even the prompting to act comes from God. For instance, you might even feel guilty, "What is this? I am sitting, idly, not doing anything. At the same time the *ashram* is feeding me, taking care of me. It's time I did something." Who makes you feel guilty? God, again. So God, in a way, asks you to do something and makes you do it; therefore, you're not responsible for it. If somebody comes and tells you something, it's not that somebody tells you; it's God telling you.

For that kind of surrender, you should have total faith in God. "Will God really take care of me if I surrender like that?" That's up to you to decide. How much faith do you have? If you really trust that way, everything will be taken care of. That's why I always say faith and fear don't go together. If you have complete faith, there's no more questioning. God will never let you down.

Sometimes you might even say, "Look at this. I trusted God, but now something is hurting me. How could God let somebody hurt me?" That's where real surrender comes: "God let that person hurt me. Okay; so why should God let him hurt me? Maybe it's for my benefit. I probably needed that experience for some reason." Sometimes, others take a patient to the hospital for an operation. The patient may not even understand that the operation will save her. In the same way, sometimes God lets you get hurt for your own benefit.

It's at that point that you need to understand that even painful events happen with God's permission. It's God who was behind it. That's where you prove that you have total faith. Of course, if everything goes nicely, everybody will have faith. But where is the proof then that you have faith? It should be tested. God will test your faith.

Let's have that complete, complete faith. Say, "God, I'm Yours. You make me act. Nothing happens to me in my life without Your doing it. And the entire universe is the same. I know You are the one who is doing everything to everybody. I realize that, too." First, realize that God is working through you always. Then, you realize that God is the same God working through everybody. If that realization comes, you are completely free from any problem, any botheration: "Everybody is equal to me. Everybody is loved by me."

May you all become that kind of realized instrument. Know that God is always working through everybody. Don't project your ego and put that label on yourself: "I did right. I did wrong." No. You couldn't do right or wrong. Just know that and let God work through you. That surrender is the biggest achievement that one can have. Let us all be good instruments. Let us know that God is functioning through us. The simple thing is to leave it to God. Be at ease. Enjoy that Supreme Love.

Necessity for a Guide

The literal meaning of Guru is teacher. But, normally, the word is used for a spiritual teacher, one who helps you in realizing your own Spirit by removing the ignorance that veils it. The word Guru is made up of two syllables–*gu* and *ru*. *Gu* means the darkness of ignorance, *ru*, the one who dispels. So, the one who dispels your ignorance is Guru.

You feel the necessity for a guide only when you don't know your way. If you know already, there's no need for a Guru. But, even in the worldly sense, we always seem to understand things through the help of somebody. For instance, when you come into the world as a baby, your mother acts as your Guru. It is she who removes the darkness with respect to knowing who your father is, and you take her word for it.

The Hindu scriptures say that everyone should have four Gurus: *Mata, Pita*, Guru, *Deva*. *Mata* is the mother; *Pita* is the father; Guru is the spiritual guide; and, ultimately, *Deva* is God. First the mother shows you the father; then the father takes you to the Guru; and, finally, the Guru takes you to God. Actually, in our normal lives, we take the help of many Gurus. When such is the case, even in the normal worldly life, how could it be otherwise in the spiritual life? Your spiritual Guru is even more necessary than the worldly ones, because the spiritual life is much more subtle.

Many people read a lot of books about Yoga and spiritual life, but books alone can never take the place of a Guru. If we could learn everything through books, then there should be only publishing houses and no universities.

Books cannot take the place of a teacher, because when you read a book, you can learn from the book, but the book can never teach you. You should know the difference. It's up to you to understand correctly what you read. The author might even have given the right meaning with all good intentions, but you read it any way you want, because you're trying to understand it with the help of your own mind, your own understanding.

The entire responsibility lies in your hands. You can understand or misunderstand. That's why we see quite a lot of misrepresentation even in the spiritual field. People read the books and then just understand or interpret as they want and even teach others that their interpretation is what Yoga is. That's why you need a person who has gone through the path and realized the goal to guide you in what's to be done. So, I would say that a spiritual teacher is very necessary.

A Guru is the one who has steady wisdom, *stithapragnyam* in Sanskrit, one who has realized the Self. Having that realization, you become so steady; you're never nervous. You'll always be tranquil; nothing can shake you. Your *pragnya* or knowledge, never fades nor gets clouded over. It's always in the Light. You call such an enlightened person *stithapragnyam*, one of steady wisdom.

It's not the body or the mind or the intellectual understanding. It's the Self that you call Guru. Only in the Self can there be perfect equanimity. It's that Divine within–not the man or woman–remember that. A person can never have this. When you see somebody and say Guru, you don't mean the physical body or his or her intelligence; you mean the Self.

That Self is in everything, in everybody, so the Guru is, also, in everything. In reality, every one of you is a Guru. But the trouble is that only some people seem to know it, and many seem not to know. We were all born with that knowledge, but, somehow, we seem to have lost it. We call this growing up–growth.

But, certainly, we know that an undesirable growth has to be operated on and removed, is it not so? And that's the business of the one whom you call a Guru. Sometimes he or she performs gentle operations, sometimes really difficult ones and sometimes with a little local anesthesia, sometimes with total anesthesia.

That steady-minded person is like the ocean: totally contented. You are a person above wants. What is meant by a person above wants? You have no wants; you never want anything. And because you don't want anything, it seems that all the things that are normally wanted by others want you.

Furthermore, no Guru is interested in creating disciples. In fact no Guru will even declare him- or herself a Guru. It's the disciples who recognize the Guru. They make a Guru. If there are no disciples, how can you call yourself a Guru? It's because a disciple learns something from someone that you call him or her a teacher.

In other words, the Guru will not make distinctions. The Guru will be totally impartial. Whether you see a sinner or saint, your eye is totally neutral–like the sun. The sun shines not only on a palace but even on a dilapidated hut or a deserted beach.

Likewise, you see that equanimity everywhere in nature. A rose will smell the same whether you've bought it, borrowed it or even if you've stolen it. It won't say, "No, no, no, you didn't buy me. You stole me from the garden. I won't give you the smell." It's only the human beings who see with these distinctions: language, skin color, caste, country. But nature, or God, has *samadarshinam*– equal vision. And that is also the quality of a steady-minded person.

Also, the Guru gets neither excited, nor depressed. You remain centered, because you have constant excitement within. There's nothing more exciting than that for you. You see everything outside as just temporary, just normal, and just fun. You're always in that intoxication from within, so nothing else can intoxicate you anymore.

In truth, you are that Guru—you are that Self. And once you realize that, you'll be possessed by all these beautiful qualities. Nothing will be able to shake you. And until that happens, nothing else can save you. So, let us realize that Self first. If you know who you are, you don't need to worry about others' opinions. Nothing affects you—pleasure or pain, praise or censure. That's the sign of a person of steady wisdom or a true devotee of God (or a Guru).

All of this is not just something intellectual. It's not that such a person makes a mental adjustment or alignment. If that were so, it would be liable to get misaligned, also. If a car runs on a bumpy road, the alignment may go wrong, and the wheels will have to be aligned again and again. So this is not mere intellectual understanding. We can first know the Self intellectually, but we should ultimately experience it. And the experience comes only when we know who we are without the slightest doubt.

Again and again, I would like to remind you not to take the physical body or even the intelligence of a teacher as the Guru. Rather, it's the Self. Because you have realized the Self, your intelligence gets a better light and your realization reflects through your intelligence. Then, that intelligence talks of something because of that experience, not because his intelligence alone is something special.

So when you address somebody as the Guru, you're addressing the Self. Let us know that positively. The scriptures say. "Guru is Lord Shiva; the Guru is Divine; the Guru is your relations; Guru is your body; Guru is your soul; Guru is your Self. There is nothing but the Guru." That means that, ultimately, everything is that Self. With a description like this, who is not the Guru? Can I say then, "I am the Guru; you are not?" No.

Everybody is the Guru. But when you don't seem to know that, you just ask me, and I say, "Hey, you are that." This is the final instruction the Guru can give a disciple when he or she is fit to understand it—simply, "You are That."

And what about the disciple? What are the qualifications of a disciple? How should one approach the Guru? You should have the sincerity and acknowledge that you know nothing (in the spiritual sense). You should not say, "I do know something; can you add a little more?" That's what you call total surrender. You accept your ignorance. Then, you're totally free from egoism. You come with a clean vessel. As long as the ego is in the vessel, whatever the Guru might put into it will get contaminated. This reminds me of a Zen story.

A disciple went to a Master to ask him for some wisdom. The Master said, "Okay, I'll give you the wisdom, but first have a cup of tea with me." Then, he began to pour the tea into the disciple's cup. And he went on pouring and pouring until the cup was overflowing. Still, he kept on pouring.

The disciple finally said, "Sir, it's already full and you're still pouring. The tea is going on the ground, not into the cup."

"Oh, I see," replied the Master. "Well, it's the same with your mind. It's already full. Whatever I say is going to overflow your cup; it can't go in. You'd better go empty your cup and, then, come back." A seeker after enlightenment should say, "I'm just empty, hollow. You are holy. Please pour that holiness into this hollowness."

Unless you have faith, you can't receive what the Guru has to give you. Devotion means that you put the entire faith in the Guru. That faith becomes your connecting link. Once that trust is established, even if the Guru refuses to teach you, you'll learn, because the power of faith is that much. By your own faith, you'll be able to understand what the Guru has in mind; he or she need not even tell you.

Without the Guru even opening the mouth, you can understand him or her, because you have established the true communication. The real teaching, or imparting of the true knowledge, is not normally done with words. We should always remember that. A Guru may give hours and hours of lectures, but it will be merely nothing compared with one minute of silent imparting. Words have their limitations, but in silence–by speaking through silence–in the proper communication, in feeling, you receive much more.

Devotion to the spiritual master is called Guru *bhakti*. But that's a very high form of *bhakti*. It's the highest one, I would say, because it's very difficult. A statue is always the same; there's never any change in it. Whenever you come, you see the same statue. It's more or less eternal–it's always God to you. But it's not so in the case of the Guru.

Sometimes, Gurus will appear to be the greatest teachers, the great Masters, the Self-realized souls; at other times, they'll be like something else. You don't always see the divine aspects. Sometimes, they might even look like devils or crazy, mad people. They are a mixture of everything. Also, Gurus won't always conform to your expectations of them. You may have your own imagination about how a Guru should be. It's because Guru worship is very difficult that it's placed above all the other forms of worship.

When it comes to choosing a Guru, you have to follow how you feel. Your heart should tell you, "Yes, so-and-so can guide me on the path." Or you can use your intelligence and question some of the students: "How is that teacher? Has he or she really taught you something?"

If you're really interested in finding a Guru, your own keen interest will show you the way. You don't need to worry about it. If you can't decide, say to yourself, "All right, I'll follow your way for some time, one or two or three months.

If nothing happens, that's all. But, if I get a little taste, then I'll know there's something there, and I'll take a little more."

Know that there is a Guru within you; there is something in you that always seems to know what's happening in you. So, as the person who knows everything, you are the Light, you are the Guru. Apply that knowledge to the things that you don't know; that is using the Guru within.

However, if you don't know how to apply your own knowing, then you go to somebody who has that capacity. The real Guru is the Spirit within you, the awareness. It is your own conscience. The conscience in you, in me, in everybody is the same. It's a part of the Cosmic Consciousness. It's the God in you that's always watching you. It can guide you and tell you whether you are doing right or wrong.

But, sometimes, we're weak and don't listen to that conscience. So, you have an outside Guru who has realized the inner Truth and who follows his or her conscience every time. That Guru helps you to know what is right and what is wrong. Even while helping you, the Guru will gradually teach you how to recognize and follow the inner Guru. True Gurus will never make you dependent on them.

Gurus are there to liberate you, not to make you dependent on them. Earlier, I said that there's not an eternal commitment to the Guru as a physical person; rather you're eternally committed to that consciousness, which is not different from your own consciousness.

Let us know that, in truth, we are the Divine image, the image of God. Somehow, the veil of our egos prevents us from realizing this. So just remove that ego. It's that ego that's the basis for all these mental dramas; it is *maya*, illusion. It creates all kinds of problems, troubles, anxieties and fears. So, please, if anybody has that ego, say "E - go!" Don't welcome it anymore. Once that goes away you become humble, and your mind will be totally under your control. You'll become the Master.

I'm not going to stipulate certain practices to achieve this; do anything you want. But see that your mind remains in that tranquility, that purity, that neutrality. No Guru can ever take some

Light and put it into you or bring God to you.
And there's no need to do that, because you have
it already. If you were to get it from the Guru,
you might lose it one day. Instead, you have it—
you are that.

The Guru only helps you to know it. You
fail to notice that Light because of the ego and
the mental disturbances that it causes. So purify
the mind; control the mind. Or, first, control the
body and the *prana* (life force) and when they are
calmed, the mind will be calmed automatically.
Then nothing can hide the Truth from you. You
become fine. If you're that fine, if you're that pure,
then you are blessed. Then, the God in you shines
out. You know that you're God, and others know
that you're God.

May that great Guru, the omnipresent Guru
who is everywhere, shine from all your being,
reflecting your refinement. That is my sincere
prayer. May that Guru express through your own
purity, humility, charity and generosity so that the
whole world could enjoy peace through you.

Understanding

Understanding is a great quality that everyone should possess. If we understand one another, we'll also understand God. Without knowing or understanding your own Self and your neighbor's Self, how are you going to understand God? When we break down the word, we see that understanding comes only when you stand under.

Some people don't want to stand under anybody. They want to be on the upper level. But humility comes only through understanding. As long as you think you're somebody special, you're not. When you realize that you're nothing special, then you really are something great. It's not an inferiority complex. It's humility. Remember, the one who has a lot of understanding is always humble.

Most likely, you're familiar with the wheat plant, and you've probably seen the wheat in the field growing straight up. As the wheat slowly grows, the tender grains are always looking up; they never bend down. But at the time when they're rich in nutrition and fully ripe, they're not straight anymore. Because there's weight in the head, they bend and bow down. An empty head will proudly stand straight up: "I'm so high!" But the mature one bends low to the ground.

That is to say, the understanding one will always be humble, and that is the greatest virtue. Wherever you see humility, there is understanding. Really, there's no limit to understanding and learning. In the Hindu faith, Saraswati, the Goddess of Wisdom, is always shown with a book in her hand, still reading. If she, herself, is still continuously learning, where is the limit?

When we are keen to learn, we won't reject anything. Actually, you don't even have to read books. If you want to know, "Ask and it shall be given." All of nature is a book of knowledge. Draw silent lessons from all around you. Listen.

The wealth of hearing is above all wealth, so always listen. You were made to listen. You were given two ears but only one mouth. That's the proof. Talk less, hear more. If you were meant to hear a word and simply accept it, then one ear would be enough, right in front. But the ears were put at the sides of your head, so that when the message comes, it should split into two halves and go on each side.

That means that you analyze it, understand it, and, only then accept it. Don't just take any word that comes as the truth. There's no door to close the ears. Those funnels that catch all the vibrations are always open, but to talk, you must pass two fences. Before a word can come out, it has to pass a row of teeth and the lips. So, keep words very sacred. Don't let them out easily. If you still want to talk, think twice.

Our understanding doesn't come only through the senses; it comes through the mind. Hearing is not enough; you have to listen. Listen with the ears and with the heart, too. There's a great difference between listening and hearing. If you listen, you need not take notes. There's a big recorder inside, multi-track, an unending tape. If you listen carefully, you're taping without any distortion.

These ideas may appear very simple, but they're the basic bricks with which to build an entire life. Without these bricks, nothing can be achieved in the spiritual area. Once, Avvaiyar, a great woman saint of South India, cried to God: "Lord, I don't know what I'm doing. I seem to have grabbed all the things from many books and learned them by heart. I seem to be talking and talking as if there were mouths all over my body. When can I get out of this and find the silence?"

Through silence you can realize the quiet witness within you. That silence is the spirit or awareness. Your awareness is silent. It never tells you anything. It's just there, simply watching you. Whether you do good or bad, right or wrong, it simply witnesses. A witness never gets involved in the case and never joins one of the sides.

God is like that, and God's creation is also like that in a way. The sun is just a witness, the wind is a witness, the sky is a witness and the water is a witness. The witness is there; that's all. In its presence, you act. And to know that silent witness that's always aware, to know the Knower, you should stop trying to know other things first.

Know other things afterward. The rest will come automatically. This may remind you of a beautiful saying in the *Bible*: Seek first the Kingdom of Heaven by which you will have everything afterward. If you don't know the Knower, even if you own the whole earth, the universe is useless to you. All the wealth you possess is just a big zero. By itself it has no value. Take a check, write a few zeros on it, and give it to somebody. He or she won't be able to get even a penny for it. Add two more zeros. Still nothing. But if you just put a one in the front and then start adding zeros, every zero will increase the value tenfold.

First, know who you are. Then, all the other knowledge will have a magnified effect. Don't forget to have that One before all your zeros. Know that you are That. Be silent and find inner knowledge. Listen to the silence. To realize, go into deep, deep silence. The only limit to wisdom is silence. In that silence realize your true nature.

There are no words to describe that Self. As the *Upanishads* say, it's not consciousness, it's not unconsciousness. It's not the sum total of all consciousness. You can't talk of it. There's no mark, no symbols. It's not located in one place. That's the essence.

A Courageous Mind

Our human capacity is limited, and even the best doctors are limited in what they can do. I'm not blaming them for it. They're doing the best they can, and they do many great things. But we know that there is another Doctor who can perform miracles. I'm not just talking about what some people might consider God, sitting somewhere apart from everything; No; I'm talking about the Cosmic Energy, the Supreme Energy, which moves every atom in this cosmos. It's that *prana*, that Energy called Parashakti, the Supreme Power.

All we have to do is to link ourselves, to open ourselves to that energy. And that will rebuild our system, however damaged it is. So, the first thing that I would like to share with you is never, never, never lose hope. Never lose hope. Because, the, moment you lose hope, that itself weakens the system a lot. It's very true.

Many of our problems are caused by the fear itself. A fearful person loses much of his or her stamina and strength. That's why my advice is: don't be afraid. Have that hope under any circumstances. That's the first way to block the drainage of vital energy; then we can fill it up again. By hope and courage, we stop draining the energy; then, we can put it back.

And that's where the natural discipline of life comes in. We call it yogic. Yoga is just leading a disciplined life, doing what is necessary to put back what we lost. All our Yoga postures, asanas, can tone our system, squeeze out the blockages, and clear the way for putting in more *prana*, vital energy. That's why, after the asanas, the *pranayama*, breathing practice, is done. I have total faith in *pranayama*. *Prana* is simple. All you have to do is take in a deep breath. It's the cheapest and the best medicine.

We should be aware of everything that we take into our system. Take food, for example. If a nice person, a loving person gives you even simple food, you enjoy it; it becomes nectar to your system. At the same time, if somebody dislikes you and serves the food to you in a disinterested way, that food immediately becomes poison in the system. So, it's not the food alone; it's the motive behind it. Don't put poison into the system. Everything is like that. It's not what you get—it's not the substance itself–it's what comes with it, what kind of vibration comes with it.

Everything that we utilize in our life should come in a gentle, loving, holy way; not contaminated, not filled with hatred, anger and fear. We have to approach this problem from various directions. It's not just one thing that created the problem, as I said earlier.

So, likewise, we have to use various approaches: spiritual approach, intellectual approach, approach through food, approach through thought, approach through society, approach through our environment. Even your room should be clean and pleasant with good vibrations. Burn some incense in your room every day. Be sure that your room is neat, that it doesn't look like a junk yard. However sick you may be, keep your surroundings neat and clean.

All these things help to heal. Remember that healing is not just one thing done by somebody else to you. You have to do certain things in order to heal. You've probably seen some rooms you can't even go into. They're torn to pieces as if ransacked by somebody. That's not a healthy thing even to look at. It won't produce good vibrations.

Also, we need to make the mind healthy and happy. Actually, we're born with that happiness, we are born with ease. But, maybe out of our ignorance, we've done something wrong to disturb the ease; and, now, we call it dis-eased. Imagine how many kinds of worries we have. How are we going to preserve our *prana*, preserve our immune system with all those worries? And how much of the worry is unwarranted? We've created a lot of worry in our minds. But take a look at that little sparrow on the tree; how happy it is. It goes, picks up something, comes back to its branch, and sits. Compare yourself to that sparrow. Let's not have all these worries.

Yes, of course there is hardship in life. I'm not saying that it doesn't exist. But worry is not going to help us in any way. You should understand that a worryless mind is very important, particularly in a situation where someone is ill. Imagine, for example, that, you have your blood tested. If the result is positive for the HIV virus, you immediately say, "Oh, I have AIDS! I don't know what to do. Am I going to die?"

When you think this way, then you're already beginning to die. So, never, never give room for that kind of thinking. Keep your mind always above the water, your head above the water. Don't let these things drown you.

In order to stay healthy and balanced, it's important to know the power of suggestion. Simply say, "No! I'm not going to die. I am just going to get out of it! I'll rebuild my system! I have strength! And I have the know-how. I will do it!" That kind of will is a great remedy that you can't get from any doctor. You have to develop it yourself. We live because we suggest that we are living. If you keep suggesting that you're dying, you will die.

Have a courageous mind. If you can't make yourself strong by your own thoughts then think that there's a greater force, God's force. That's where faith comes in: "I have my faith in God. I am God's child. God is not going to let me down. I might have made mistakes. I feel sorry for it. I'm changing all those things, changing my lifestyle. And God is going to help me." Faith moves mountains. Faith the size of a mustard seed can blow the mountains apart. You are what you believe in.

A Better World

Who creates war? The bombs don't drop
by themselves. It's the people behind them, the
human minds that create war. If we want peace,
where should we begin? With the minds of the
people. If the minds are changed, the world will
change. There's a saying: "As the man, so the
world; as the mind, so the man." Change the mind,
you change the person; and change the person,
you change the community or the society or the
nation or the world.

If you can't have communion with your own
neighbor, how are you going to have communion
with God? Your neighbor is God in a visible form.
Let us have communion with our own neighbors—
next door and around the globe.

We need to use the spiritual teachings of
whatever faith we choose to help us have real love
for one another. Even war is based on love, but
that love is misplaced or limited in some way. If
you want to throw a bomb on another country,
you may feel that you're doing it for the sake of
your country, because you love your country. All
right, you should love your country, but don't you

think the other person will love his or her own country in the same way? If your love is universal, how can you bomb someone else? Those people are your brothers and sisters.

The whole world is like a body. If not treated, an infection in one part will spread throughout the whole body. Every part will be affected. Likewise, if we want to be happy, we should work for the happiness of all people everywhere. That is the only way to achieve real peace and contentment. Unless the human mind is freed from greed, jealousy and hatred, there will be more and more wars.

If you free your own mind of all these problems, at least that little part of the world will be free from trouble. If we want a world free from violence, we should free ourselves from every kind of violence, even in thought. If we want a peaceful world, let us begin with ourselves. If we want peace outside, we must have it within first.

I consider this a transitory period. We are witnessing a great change. When a seedling is transplanted, at first its leaves wither and fall. It has to face that stage; that's part of the process of getting rooted in the earth. The seedling can't live in the nursery always. In the same way, I see a very bright future for humankind; we are slowly getting rooted. This, itself, is the proof of what's to come. I really feel that we're going to see a better world. May that universal love light our paths.

May the whole world be filled with peace and joy, love and light.

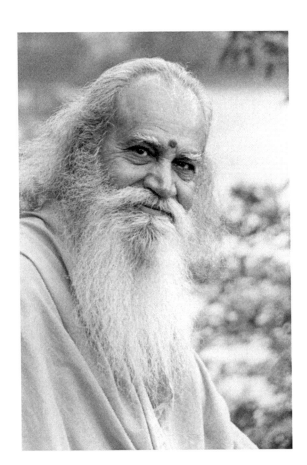

Sri Swami Satchidananda

Sri Swami Satchidananda was one of the first Yoga masters to bring the classical Yoga tradition to the West. He taught Yoga postures to Americans, introduced them to meditation, vegetarian diet and a more compassionate lifestyle.

During this period of cultural awakening, iconic pop artist Peter Max and a small circle of his artist friends beseeched the Swami to extend his brief stop in New York City so they could learn from him the secret of finding physical, mental and spiritual health, peace and enlightenment.

Three years later, he led some half a million American youth in chanting *OM*, when he delivered the official opening remarks at the 1969 Woodstock Music and Art Festival and he became known as "the Woodstock Guru."

The distinctive teachings he brought with him blend the physical discipline of Yoga, the spiritual philosophy of Vedantic literature and the interfaith ideals he pioneered.

These techniques and concepts influenced a generation and spawned a Yoga culture that is flourishing today. Today, over twenty million Americans practice Yoga as a means for managing stress, promoting health, slowing down the aging process and creating a more meaningful life.

The teachings of Swami Satchidananda have spread into the mainstream and thousands of people now teach Yoga. Integral Yoga is the foundation for Dr. Dean Ornish's landmark work in reversing heart disease and Dr. Michael Lerner's noted Commonweal Cancer Help program.

Today, Integral Yoga Institutes, teaching centers and certified teachers throughout the United States and abroad offer classes and training programs in all aspects of Integral Yoga.

In 1979, Sri Swamiji was inspired to establish Satchidananda Ashram–Yogaville. Based on his teachings, it is a place where people of different faiths and backgrounds can come to realize their essential oneness.

One of the focal points of Yogaville is the Light Of Truth Universal Shrine (LOTUS). This unique interfaith shrine honors the Spirit that unites all the world religions, while celebrating their diversity. People from all over the world come there to meditate and pray.

Over the years, Sri Swamiji received many honors for his public service, including the Juliet Hollister Interfaith Award presented at the United Nations and in 2002 the U Thant Peace Award.

In addition, he served on the advisory boards of many Yoga, world peace and interfaith organizations. He is the author of many books on Yoga and is the subject of the documentary, *Living Yoga: The life and teachings of Swami Satchidananda.*

In 2002, he entered *Mahasamadhi* (a God-realized soul's conscious final exit from the body).

For more information, visit: www.swamisatchidananda.org